MW00509510

# Sirtfood diet for beginners

The ultimate recipe guide starts to lose weight fast, reset metabolism, lower blood pressure and more. Very suitable for busy people and beginners

**SOPHIE GARDNER**

# Sommario

# INTRODUCTION

Theoretically, this slimming diet is sold to make you lose weight quickly and without depriving yourself. It appeared for the first time in 2016 in a book soberly entitled The Sirtfood diet and written by two English graduates in nutritional medicine, Aidan Goggins and then Glen Matten.

In practice, this involves consuming "superfoods" that are sirtuins rich, belonging to a family of enzymes with seven members, for example, SIRT1, SIRT2, up to SIRT7. According to the authors, these enzymes with multiple benefits boost the immune system; it protects against neurodegenerative diseases and can act against cell aging.

Among the foods that would contain these famous enzymes are apples, blueberries, coffee, matcha tea, turmeric, dates, celery, onion, citrus, olive oil, arugula, soy, but also dark chocolate and red wine!

The Sirtuin Diet (in the original Sirtfood Diet) is based on proteins. But she still has nothing in common with Low-Carb, Paleo & Co. Because, as the name suggests, the focus is on an exceptional protein - the enzyme Sirtuin. Anyone who has thought directly of animal products when it comes to proteins is wrong.

They are plant foods that stimulate the formation of the enzyme and form the nutritional form's basic idea. A new era of superfoods. And something else distinguishes the trend from all the others: long-term calories do not have to be counted, nor are certain foods prohibited.

The idea: inclusion instead of exclusion

The diet was developed by the British nutritionists Aidan Goggins and Glen Matten. Their theory: The enzyme that is particularly active in lean of people and fat loss. This can be stimulated by eating certain foods.

Sirtuins are also released during fasting, but the inventors wanted to avoid the negative side effects of a strict fasting cure.

Kick start for the metabolism

In the beginning, a 2-phase diet is recommended to fuel the metabolism and the sirtuins. One thousand calories are consumed in the first three days. After that, the intake is increased to 1500 calories. Here you stick to green juices and sirtuin-based meals.

After seven days you eat again as needed, of course still a potpourri of sirt foods. These phases are not a must! Even if you "only" integrate the sirt foods and live healthily, you will see success.

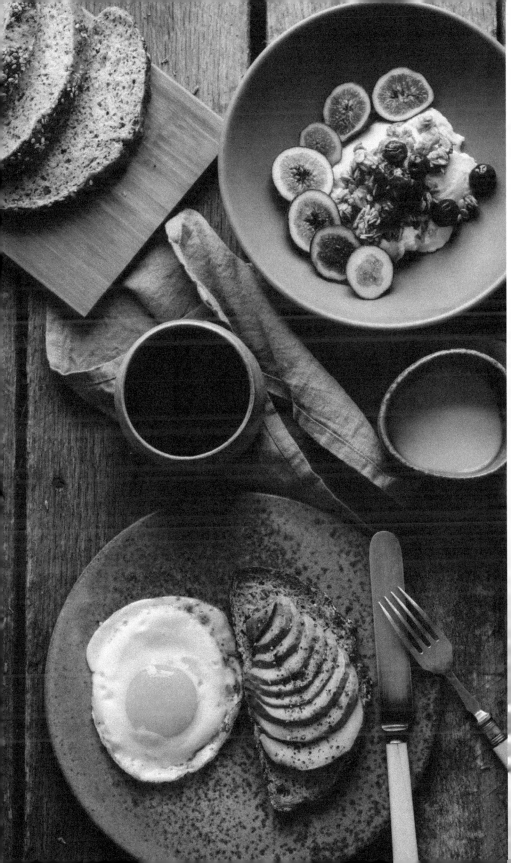

# SIRTFOOD BREAKFAST

# Ultimate Chocolate Chip Cookie N' Oreo Fudge Brownie Bar

**Preparation Time:** 30 minutes

**Cooking Time:** 30 minutes

**Servings:** 4

**Ingredients:**

- 1 cup (2 sticks) butter, softened
- 1 cup granulated sugar
- 3/4 cup light brown sugar
- 2 big eggs
- 1 tablespoon pure vanilla extract
- 2 1/2 cups all-purpose flour
- 1 tsp baking soda
- 1 tsp lemon
- 2 cups (12 oz) milk chocolate chips
- Inch packaging double stuffed Oreos
- Inch family-size (9×1 3) brownie mixture
- 1/4 cup hot fudge topping

**Directions:**

1. Preheat oven to 350 degrees f.
2. Cream the butter and sugars in a large bowl using an electric mixer at medium speed for 35 minutes.

3. Add the vanilla and eggs and mix well to combine thoroughly. In another bowl, whisk together the flour, baking soda and salt, and slowly incorporate it in the mixer till the bread is simply connected.

4. Stir in chocolate chips.

5. Spread the cookie dough at the bottom of a 9×1-3 baking dish that is wrapped with wax paper and then coated with cooking spray.

6. Shirt with a coating of Oreos. Mix brownie mix, adding an optional 1/4 cup of hot fudge directly into the mixture.

7. Twist the brownie batter within the cookie-dough and Oreos.

8. Cover with foil and bake at 350 degrees f for half an hour.

9. Remove foil and continue baking for another 15-25 minutes.

10. Let cool before cutting on brownies might nevertheless be gooey at the midst while warm, but will also place up ideally once chilled.

**Nutrition:** Calories 483 Fat 25g Carbohydrates 63g Protein 5g

# Crunchy Chocolate Chip Coconut Macadamia Nut Cookies

**Preparation Time: 30 minutes**

**Cooking Time: 3 minutes**

**Servings: 4**

**Ingredients:**

- 1 cup yogurt
- 1 cup yogurt
- 1/2 tsp baking soda
- 1/2 tsp salt
- 1 tbsp. of butter, softened
- 1 cup firmly packed brown sugar
- 1/2 cup sugar
- 1 big egg
- 1/2 cup semi-sweet chocolate chips
- 1/2 cup sweetened flaked coconut
- 1/2 cup coarsely chopped dry-roasted macadamia nuts
- 1/2 cup craisins

**Directions:**

1. Preheat the oven to 325°f.
2. In a little bowl, whisk together the flour, oats and baking soda and salt, then place aside.

3. On your mixer bowl, then mix the butter/ sugar/egg mix.

4. Mix from the flour/oats mix until just combined and stir into the chocolate chips, craisins, nuts, and coconut.

5. Outsized bits on a parchment-lined cookie sheet.

6. Bake for 1-3 minutes before biscuits are only barely golden brown.

7. Remove from the oven and then leave the cookie sheets to cool at least 10 minutes.

**Nutrition:** Calories 616 Fat 35g Carbohydrates 82g Protein 5g

# Blueberry Muffins

**Preparation Time:** 15 Minutes

**Cooking Time:** 20 Minutes

**Servings:** 8

**Ingredients:**

- 1 cup buckwheat flour
- ¼ cup arrowroot starch
- 1½ teaspoons baking powder
- ¼ teaspoon sea salt
- 2 eggs
- ½ cup unsweetened almond milk
- 2–3 tablespoons maple syrup
- 2 tablespoons coconut oil, melted
- 1 cup fresh blueberries

**Directions:**

1. Preheat your oven to 350°F and line 8 cups of a muffin tin.
2. In a bowl, place the buckwheat flour, arrowroot starch, baking powder, and salt, and mix well.
3. In a separate bowl, place the eggs, almond milk, maple syrup, and coconut oil, and beat until well combined.
4. Now, place the flour mixture and mix until just combined.
5. Gently, fold in the blueberries.

6. Transfer the mixture into prepared muffin cups evenly.

7. Bake for about 25 minutes or until a toothpick inserted in the center comes out clean.

8. Remove the muffin tin from oven and place onto a wire rack to cool for about 10 minutes.

9. Carefully invert the muffins onto the wire rack to cool completely before serving.

**Nutrition:** Calories 136 Fat 5.3 g Carbs 20.7 g Protein 3.5 g

# Chocolate Waffles

**Preparation Time: 15 Minutes**

**Cooking Time: 24 Minutes**

**Servings: 8**

**Ingredients:**

- 2 cups unsweetened almond milk
- 1 tablespoon fresh lemon juice
- 1 cup buckwheat flour
- ½ cup cacao powder
- ¼ cup flaxseed meal
- 1 teaspoon baking soda
- 1 teaspoon baking powder
- ¼ teaspoons kosher salt
- 2 large eggs
- ½ cup coconut oil, melted
- ¼ cup dark brown sugar
- 2 teaspoons vanilla extract
- 2 ounces unsweetened dark chocolate, chopped roughly

**Directions:**

1. In a bowl, add the almond milk and lemon juice and mix well.

___

2. Set aside for about 10 minutes.

3. In a bowl, place buckwheat flour, cacao powder, flaxseed meal, baking soda, baking powder, and salt, and mix well.

4. In the bowl of almond milk mixture, place the eggs, coconut oil, brown sugar, and vanilla extract, and beat until smooth.

5. Now, place the flour mixture and beat until smooth.

6. Gently, fold in the chocolate pieces.

7. Preheat the waffle iron and then grease it.

8. Place the desired amount of the mixture into the preheated waffle iron and cook for about 3 minutes, or until golden-brown.

9. Repeat with the remaining mixture.

**Nutrition:** Calories 295 Fat 22.1 g Carbs 1.5 g Protein 6.3 g

# Salmon & Kale Omelet

**Preparation Time: 10 Minutes**

**Cooking Time: 7 Minutes**

**Servings: 4**

**Ingredients:**

- 6 eggs
- 2 tablespoons unsweetened almond milk
- Salt and ground black pepper, to taste
- 2 tablespoons olive oil
- 4 ounces smoked salmon, cut into bite-sized chunks
- 2 cup fresh kale, tough ribs removed and chopped finely
- 4 scallions, chopped finely

**Directions:**

1. In a bowl, place the eggs, coconut milk, salt, and black pepper, and beat well. Set aside.
2. In a non-stick wok, heat the oil over medium heat.
3. Place the egg mixture evenly and cook for about 30 seconds, without stirring.
4. Place the salmon kale and scallions on top of egg mixture evenly.

5. Now, reduce heat to low.

6. With the lid, cover the wok and cook for about 4–5 minutes, or until omelet is done completely.

7. Uncover the wok and cook for about 1 minute.

8. Carefully, transfer the omelet onto a serving plate and serve.

**Nutrition:** Calories 210 Fat 14.9 g Carbs 5.2 g Protein 14.8 g

# Moroccan Spiced Eggs

**Preparation Time: 60 Minutes**

**Cooking Time: 50 Minutes**

**Servings: 2**

**Ingredients:**

- 1 tsp olive oil

- One shallot, stripped and finely hacked

- One red (chime) pepper, deseeded and finely hacked

- One garlic clove, stripped and finely hacked

- One courgette (zucchini), stripped and finely hacked

- 1 tbsp tomato puree (glue)

- ½ tsp gentle stew powder

- ¼ tsp ground cinnamon

- ¼ tsp ground cumin

- ½ tsp salt

- 400g (14oz) can hacked tomatoes

- 400g (14oz) may chickpeas in water

- a little bunch of level leaf parsley (10g (1/3oz)), cleaved

- Four medium eggs at room temperature

**Directions:**

1. Heat the oil in a pan, include the shallot and red (ringer) pepper and fry delicately for 5 minutes. At that point include the garlic and courgette (zucchini) and cook for one more moment or two. Include the tomato puree (glue), flavours and salt and mix through.

2. Add the cleaved tomatoes and chickpeas (dousing alcohol and all) and increment the warmth to medium. With the top of the dish, stew the sauce for 30 minutes – ensure it is delicately rising all through and permit it to lessen in volume by around 33%.

3. Remove from the warmth and mix in the cleaved parsley.

4. Preheat the grill to 200C/180C fan/350F.

5. When you are prepared to cook the eggs, bring the tomato sauce up to a delicate stew and move to a little broiler confirmation dish.

6. Crack the eggs on the dish and lower them delicately into the stew. Spread with thwart and prepare in the grill for 10-15 minutes. Serve the blend in unique dishes with the eggs coasting on the top.

**Nutrition:** Calories: 116 Protein: 6.97 g Fat: 5.22 g Carbohydrates: 13.14 g

# Chilaquiles with Gochujang

**Preparation Time: 30 Minutes**

**Cooking Time: 20 Minutes**

**Servings: 2**

**Ingredients:**

- One dried ancho chili

- 2 cups of water

- 1 cup squashed tomatoes

- Two cloves of garlic

- One teaspoon genuine salt

- ½ tablespoons gochujang

- 5 to 6 cups tortilla chips

- Three enormous eggs

- One tablespoon olive oil

**Directions:**

1. Get the water to heat a pot. I cheated marginally and heated the water in an electric pot and emptied it into the pan. There's no sound unrivalled strategy here. Add the anchor Chile to the bubbled water and drench for 15 minutes to give it an opportunity to stout up.

2. When completed, use tongs or a spoon to extricate Chile. Make sure to spare the water for the sauce!

---

Nonetheless, on the off chance that you incidentally dump the water, it's not the apocalypse.

3. Mix the doused Chile, 1 cup of saved high temp water, squashed tomatoes, garlic, salt and gochujang until smooth.

4. Empty sauce into a large dish and warmth over medium warmth for 4 to 5 minutes. Mood killer the heat and include the tortilla chips. Mix the chips to cover with the sauce. In a different skillet, shower a teaspoon of oil and fry an egg on top, until the whites have settled. Plate the egg and cook the remainder of the eggs. If you are phenomenal at performing various tasks, you can likely sear the eggs while you heat the red sauce. I am not precisely so capable.

5. Top the chips with the seared eggs, cotija, hacked cilantro, jalapeños, onions and avocado. Serve right away.

**Nutrition:** Calories: 484 kcal Protein: 14.55 g Fat: 18.62 g Carbohydrates: 64.04 g

# Twice Baked Breakfast Potatoes

**Preparation Time: 1 hour 10 Minutes**

**Cooking Time: 60 Minutes**

**Servings: 2**

**Ingredients:**

- 2 medium reddish brown potatoes, cleaned and pricked with a fork everywhere
- 2 tablespoons unsalted spread
- 3 tablespoons overwhelming cream
- 4 rashers cooked bacon
- 4 huge eggs
- ½ cup destroyed cheddar
- Daintily cut chives
- Salt and pepper to taste

**Directions:**

1. Preheat grill to 400°F.
2. Spot potatoes straightforwardly on stove rack in the focal point of the grill and prepare for 30 to 45 min.
3. Evacuate and permit potatoes to cool for around 15 minutes.

4. Cut every potato down the middle longwise and burrow every half out, scooping the potato substance into a blending bowl.

5. Gather margarine and cream to the potato and pound into a single unit until smooth — season with salt and pepper and mix.

6. Spread a portion of the potato blend into the base of each emptied potato skin and sprinkle with one tablespoon cheddar (you may make them remain pounded potato left to snack on).

7. Add one rasher bacon to every half and top with a raw egg.

8. Spot potatoes onto a heating sheet and come back to the appliance.

9. Lower broiler temperature to 375°F and heat potatoes until egg whites simply set and yolks are as yet runny.

10. Top every potato with a sprinkle of the rest of the cheddar, season with salt and pepper and finish with cut chives.

**Nutrition:** Calories: 647 kcal Protein: 30.46 g Fat: 55.79 g Carbohydrates: 7.45 g

# Sirt Muesli

**Preparation Time:** 30 Minutes

**Cooking Time:** 0 Minutes

**Servings:** 2

**Ingredients:**

- 20g (¾ oz.) buckwheat drops
- 10g (⅜ oz.) buckwheat puffs
- 15g (½ oz.) coconut drops or dried up coconut
- 40g (1 ½ oz.) Medjool dates, hollowed and slashed
- 15g (½ oz.) pecans, slashed
- 10g (⅜ oz.) cocoa nibs
- 100g (3 ½ oz.) strawberries, hulled and slashed
- 100g (3 ½ oz.) plain Greek yoghurt (or vegetarian elective, for example, soya or coconut yoghurt)

**Directions:**

1. Blend the entirety of the above fixings (forget about the strawberries and yoghurt if not serving straight away).

**Nutrition:** Calories: 334 kcal Protein: 4.39 g Fat: 22.58 g Carbohydrates: 34.35 g

# Mushroom Scramble Eggs

**Preparation Time: 45 Minutes**

**Cooking Time: 10 Minutes**

**Servings: 2**

**Ingredients:**

- 2 eggs

- 1 tsp ground turmeric

- 1 tsp mellow curry powder

- 20g (¾ oz.) kale, generally slashed

- 1 tsp additional virgin olive oil

- ½ superior bean stew, daintily cut

- Bunch of catch mushrooms, meagerly cut

- 5g (3/16oz.) parsley, finely slashed

- *Optional* Add a seed blend as a topper and some Rooster Sauce for enhance

**Directions:**

1. Blend the turmeric and curry powder and include a little water until you have accomplished a light glue.

2. Steam the kale for 2–3 minutes.

3. Warmth the oil in a skillet over medium heat and fry the bean stew and mushrooms for 2–3 minutes until they have begun to darker and mollify.

4. Include the eggs and flavour glue and cook over a medium warmth at that point add the kale and keep on cooking over medium heat for a further moment. At long last, include the parsley, blend well and serve.

**Nutrition:** Calories: 158 kcal Protein: 9.96 g Fat: 10.93 g Carbohydrates: 5.04 g

# Smoked Salmon Omelets

**Preparation Time: 45 Minutes**

**Cooking Time: 15 Minutes**

**Servings: 2**

**Ingredients:**

- 2 Medium eggs
- 100 g (3 ½ oz.) Smoked salmon, cut
- 1/2 tsp Capers
- 10 g (⅜ oz.) Rocket, slashed
- 1 tsp Parsley, slashed
- 1 tsp extra virgin olive oil

**Directions:**

1. Split the eggs into a bowl and whisk well. Include the salmon, tricks, rocket and parsley. Warmth the olive oil in a non-stick skillet until hot yet not smoking. Include the egg blend and, utilizing a spatula or fish cut, move the mixture around the dish until it is even. Diminish the warmth and let the omelette cook through. Slide the spatula around the edges and move up or crease the omelette fifty-fifty to serve.

**Nutrition:** Calories: 148 kcal Protein: 15.87 g Fat: 8.73 g Carbohydrates: 0.36 g

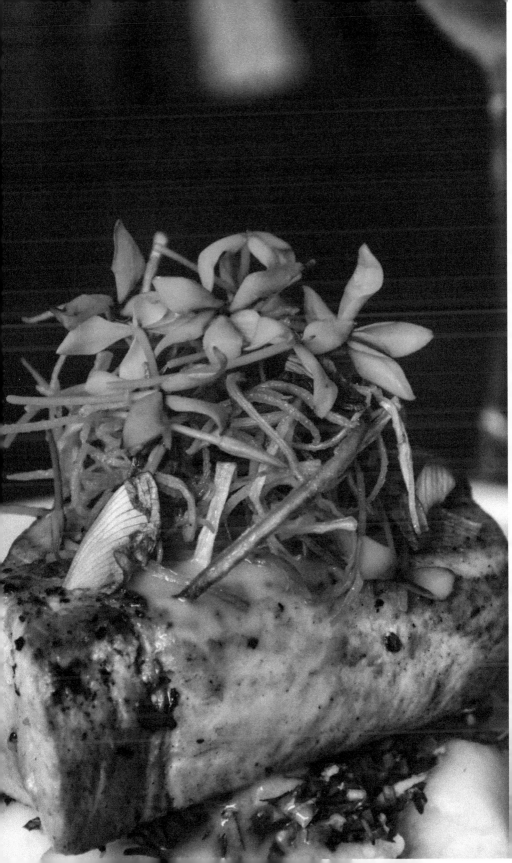

# SIRTFOOD LUNCH

# Slow Cooker Bone Broth

**Preparation Time: 5 minutes**

**Cooking Time: 24 hours**

**Servings: 16**

**Ingredients:**

- 3 pounds of assorted animal bones, with marrow

- 1 gallon of water

- 3 tablespoons salt

- 2 tablespoons ground black pepper

**Directions:**

1. Add assorted bones to a slow cooker. Pour in the water and season with salt and pepper. Turn the slow cooker to high.

2. Bring the water inside the slow cooker to a boil. This may take up to 20 minutes due to the large amount of water. Then reduce the temperature settings to low and allow to simmer for up to 24 hours. Letting the bone broth cook for this long gives you a more nutritious and tastier product. You do not need to stir the broth during this time. If necessary, add more water around the 12-hour mark if you notice the water level has dropped far below the top of the bones.

3. Shut off the heat and let the broth cool. Strain into a large stockpot or other container and discard the remains of the bones. Enjoy hot or allow to cool completely before packaging for refrigeration or freezing. The bone broth will solidify in the fridge, so simply reheat leftovers.

**Nutrition:** Calories: 56 Total fat: 2 g Sodium: 480 mg Total carbohydrates: 0 g Fiber: 0 g Sugar: 0 g Protein: 9 g

# Chicken Broth

**Preparation Time:** 5 minutes

**Cooking Time:** 150 minutes

**Servings:** 12

**Ingredients:**

- 2 pounds chicken bones, any kind
- ½ pound chicken paws
- 2 liters water
- 2 tablespoons salt
- 1 tablespoon ground black pepper

**Directions:**

1. Add chicken bones and chicken paws to the pressure cooker. Pour in water and add salt and pepper. Do not exceed about one inch below the maximum fill line.

2. Use the sealing ring to lock the lid in place and turn the steam release knob to sealing. Set the pressure cooker to high pressure for two hours.

3. After two hours have passed, allow the pressure to release, which should take about 20 minutes. Allow the broth to cool a bit, then strain into a stockpot or other large container. Enjoy hot or transfer to an appropriate

container to refrigerate or freeze. Reheat when you are ready to use.

**Nutrition:** Calories: 48 Total fat: 2 g Sodium: 520 mg Total carbohydrates: 0 g Fiber: 0 g Sugar: 0 g Protein: 7 g

# Garlic Chicken

**Preparation Time:** 5 minutes

**Cooking Time:** 20 minutes

**Servings:** 4

**Ingredients:**

- 1 ½ pounds chicken thighs
- 2 tablespoons grass-fed butter
- 1 tablespoon garlic powder
- 1 teaspoon pink Himalayan sea salt
- ½ teaspoon ground black pepper

**Directions:**

1. Season chicken thighs with garlic powder, sea salt, and black pepper. The chicken should be fairly well coated with garlic powder, so feel free to add more if necessary.

2. Melt butter in a skillet over medium-high heat. Add chicken thighs to the pan skin-side down, two thighs at a time. This is to prevent overcrowding, which can cause the chicken to become soggy.

3. Cook chicken for six minutes, shifting the chicken thighs around occasionally to prevent sticking and burning.

4. Flip chicken thighs and cook for eight minutes on the opposite side. Then flip once more and cook for another two to four minutes, or until the outside of the chicken has reached a golden brown on both sides and the skin has become crispy. Plate and serve.

**Nutrition:** Calories: 321 Total fat: 22 g Sodium: 651 mg Total carbohydrates: 1 g Fiber: 1 g Sugar: 1 g Protein: 31 g

# Bacon-wrapped Chicken

**Preparation Time:** 5 minutes

**Cooking Time:** 25 minutes

**Servings:** 4

**Ingredients:**

- 2 ½ pounds chicken breasts

- 8 slices bacon

- 1 teaspoon garlic powder

- ½ teaspoon ground black pepper

**Directions:**

1. Preheat oven to 350 degrees Fahrenheit.

2. Season chicken breasts with garlic powder and black pepper. Wrap chicken breasts in two slices of bacon each so that they are completely covered. Stick one or two toothpicks through each breast to hold the bacon in place.

3. Line a deep baking dish with aluminum foil. Arrange chicken on the baking sheet to avoid overlap and give each piece of chicken as much space as possible.

4. Transfer baking dish to the oven and cook for about 25 minutes. The bacon around the exterior of the chicken should be crisp, and the interior should have no pink

remaining when cut open. If pink remains, return chicken to the oven for an additional three to four minutes.

**Nutrition:** Calories: 309 Total fat: 12 g Sodium: 476 mg Total carbohydrates: 1 g Fiber: 1 g Sugar: 0 g Protein: 45 g

# Shredded Chicken

**Preparation Time:** 5 minutes

**Cooking Time:** 40 minutes

**Servings:** 4

**Ingredients:**

- 1 ½ pounds chicken thighs
- 1 cup homemade bone broth or chicken broth
- 2 teaspoons garlic powder
- ½ teaspoon pink Himalayan sea salt
- ½ teaspoon ground black pepper

**Directions:**

1. Preheat oven to 350 degrees Fahrenheit.

2. Add chicken thighs, garlic powder, salt, and pepper to a large pot. Combine with warmed bone broth or chicken broth, and fill the rest of the pot with water until chicken thighs are covered.

3. Bring to a boil over medium-high heat, then reduce heat to low and let simmer for about 30 minutes. The chicken should be tender enough to be easily pierced by a fork and provide little resistance.

4. Move chicken to a cutting board or other clean flat surface. Do not discard the leftover broth, as you will use it later.

5. Using two forks or a pair of meat shredder claws, pull the chicken apart into thin shreds. If using a pair of forks, use one fork to stabilize the chicken thigh and the other to shred the chicken by inserting it near the first fork and pulling away towards the edge of the thigh. If using shredder claws, simply pull both claws away from each other until all meat has been shredded.

6. Line a baking sheet with aluminum foil or parchment paper. Spread the shredded chicken out across the surface and drizzle about half a cup of the broth from the pot over top. Put the baking sheet in the oven and cook for around 10 minutes so that the chicken is slightly crispy and ready to serve.

**Nutrition:** Calories: 294 Total fat: 18 g Sodium: 542 mg Total carbohydrates: 1 g Fiber: 1 g Sugar: 1 g Protein: 34 g

# Chicken with Red Onion and Kale

Preparation Time: 15 minutes

Cooking Time: 40 minutes

Servings: 2

Ingredients:

- 120 g chicken breast
- 130 g of tomatoes
- 1 Bird's Eye chili
- 1 tablespoon of capers
- 5 g of parsley
- Lemon juice
- 2 teaspoons of extra virgin olive oil
- 2 teaspoons of turmeric
- 50 g of kale
- 20 g of red onion
- 1 teaspoon fresh ginger
- 50 g of buckwheat

Directions:

1. Marinate the chicken breast for 10 minutes with 1/4 of lemon juice, 1 teaspoon of extra virgin olive oil and 1 teaspoon of turmeric powder. Cut 130 g of tomatoes into chunks, remove the inside, season with the chili

pepper, 1 tablespoon of capers, 1 teaspoon of turmeric and one of extra virgin olive oil, 1/4 lemon juice and 5 g of chopped parsley.

2. Cook the drained chicken breast on high heat for one minute per side and then put it in the oven for about 10 minutes, at 220 °. Let it rest covered by an aluminum foil. Steam the minced kale for 5 minutes, in a pan fry the red onion, a teaspoon of grated fresh ginger and a teaspoon of extra virgin olive oil; add the boiled cabbage and leave to flavor for one minute on the fire, boil the buckwheat with the turmeric, drain and serve with the chicken, tomatoes and chopped kale.

**Nutrition:** Calories: 305 Carbohydrates: 10g Fat: 12g Protein: 37g

# Turkey with Cauliflower Couscous

**Preparation Time:** 15 minutes

**Cooking Time:** 40 minutes

**Servings:** 3

**Ingredients:**

- 150 g of turkey
- 150 g of cauliflower
- 40 g of red onion
- 1 teaspoon fresh ginger
- 1 pepper Bird's Eye
- 1 clove of garlic
- 3 tablespoons of extra virgin olive oil
- 2 teaspoons of turmeric
- 30 g of dried tomatoes
- 10 g parsley
- Dried sage to taste
- 1 tablespoon of capers
- 1/4 of fresh lemon juice

**Directions:**

1. Blend the raw cauliflower tops and cook them in a teaspoon of extra virgin olive oil, garlic, red onion, chili pepper, ginger, and a teaspoon of turmeric.

2. Leave to flavor on the fire for a minute, then add the chopped sun-dried tomatoes and 5 g of parsley. Season the turkey slice with a teaspoon of extra virgin olive oil, the dried sage and cook it in another teaspoon of extra virgin olive oil. Once ready, season with a tablespoon of capers, 1/4 of lemon juice, 5 g of parsley, a tablespoon of water and add the cauliflower.

**Nutrition:** Calories: 200 Fat: 3g Cholesterol: 70mg Sodium: 310mg Carbohydrates: 6g Protein: 30g

# Oriental Prawns with Buckwheat

**Preparation Time:** 5 minutes

**Cooking Time:** 15 minutes

**Servings:** 4

**Ingredients:**

- 150g of shrimps
- 1 spoon of turmeric
- 1 spoon of extra-virgin oil
- 75 gr of grain spaghetti
- Cooking water
- Salt
- 1 clove of garlic
- Bird's Eye chili
- 1 spoon of ginger
- Red onion
- 40 g of celery
- 75 g of green beans
- 50 g of kale
- Broth

**Directions:**

1. Cook for 2-3 minutes the peeled prawns with 1 teaspoon of tamari and 1 teaspoon of extra virgin olive oil. Boil the buckwheat noodles in salt-free water, drain and set aside.

2. Fry with another teaspoon of extra virgin olive oil, 1 clove of garlic, 1 Bird's Eye chili and 1 teaspoon of finely chopped fresh ginger, 20 g of red onion and 40 g of sliced celery, 75 g of chopped green beans, 50 g of curly kale roughly chopped.

3. Add 100 ml of broth and bring to a boil, letting it simmer until the vegetables are cooked and soft. Add the prawns, spaghetti, and 5 g of celery leaves, bring to the boil, and serve.

**Nutrition:** Calories: 180 Carbohydrates: 18g Fat: 18g Protein: 12g

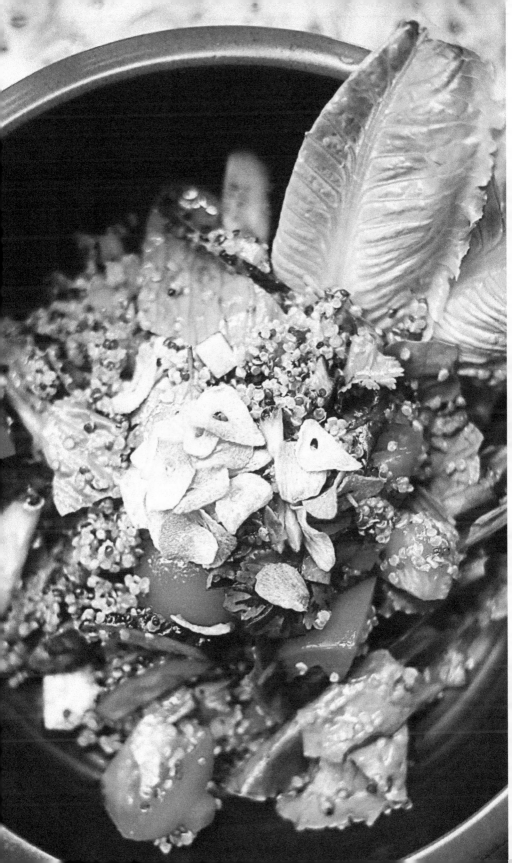

# SIRTFOOD DINNER

# Turkey Mole Tacos

**Preparation Time:** 10 minutes

**Cooking Time:** 15 minutes

**Servings:** 3

**Ingredients:**

- 75 pound lean ground turkey
- 4 stalks green onion, chopped
- 2 garlic cloves, minced
- 1 rib celery, chopped
- 3.5 ounces roasted sweet peppers, chopped and drained
- 7 ounces diced tomatoes
- 6 corn tortillas 6 inches
- 1 red onion, thinly sliced
- 2 tablespoons walnuts, roasted, chopped
- 2 ounces dark chocolate, chopped
- .25 teaspoon sea salt
- 4 teaspoons chili powder
- .5 teaspoon cumin
- .125 teaspoon ground cinnamon,

**Directions:**

1. In a large skillet that is non-stick cook the ground turkey with the green onions, celery, and garlic over medium heat. Cook until there is no pink remaining, the turkey has reached a temperature of one-hundred and sixty-five degrees, and the vegetables are tender.

2. Into the skillet with the cooked turkey add the canned tomatoes, roasted red peppers, cinnamon, chocolate, chili powder, cumin, and sea salt. Allow the liquid from the tomatoes to come to a boil before reducing the heat to medium-low, covering the skillet with a lid, and simmering for ten minutes. Stir occasionally to prevent sticking and burning.

3. Remove the cooked ground turkey from the heat and stir in the walnuts.

4. Divide the taco meat between the corn tortillas, topping it off with the sliced red onion. Serve while warm.

**Nutrition:** Calories: 475 Fat: 3g Cholesterol: 70mg Sodium: 310mg Carbohydrates: 6g Protein: 30g

# Sweet and Sour Tofu

**Preparation Time: 10 minutes**

**Cooking Time: 15 minutes**

**Servings: 4**

**Ingredients:**

- Tofu, firm – 14 ounces

- Cornstarch – 8 tablespoons, divided

- Egg white – 1

- Pineapple, chopped – 1 cup

- Bell pepper, chopped – 2

- Rice vinegar – 6 tablespoons

- Date sugar – 6 tablespoons

- Tamari sauce – 2 tablespoons

- Sea salt – 1 teaspoon

- Tomato paste – 2 tablespoons

- Water – 2 teaspoons

- Cornstarch – 2 tablespoons

- Sesame seeds, toasted – 1 teaspoon

**Directions:**

1. Line an aluminum baking sheet with kitchen parchment or a silicone sheet and set the oven to Fahrenheit three-hundred and fifty degrees.

2. Begin by pressing your tofu and then slicing it into bite-sized cubes. Sprinkle two of the eight divided tablespoons of cornstarch over the tofu, tossing it until the tofu is evenly coated.

3. Place the remaining six tablespoons of divided cornstarch in one bowl and the egg white (or aquafaba) in another.

4. Dip a few tofu cubes at a time first in the egg white and then in the cornstarch. Transfer the breaded cubes to the prepared baking sheet and continue the process until all the cubes are prepared. Arrange the tofu cubes on the pan evenly so that they don't touch, and then bake until crispy, about fifteen to twenty minutes.

5. While the tofu cooks, whisk together the rice vinegar, date sugar, tamari sauce, sea salt, tomato paste, water, two tablespoons of corn starch, and the sesame seeds.

6. Add the peppers and pineapple to a large skillet and sauté them until slightly tender. Add in the mixed sauce and deglaze the skillet. Add the cooked tofu to the skillet and continue to cook it in the sauce until it is coated and sticky and the sauce has thickened.

7. Serve while warm over brown rice or buckwheat.

**Nutrition:** Calories: 366

# BBQ Tempeh Sandwiches

**Preparation Time:** 15 minutes

**Cooking Time:** 40 minutes

**Servings:** 4

**Ingredients:**

- Tempeh, sliced into long strips – 8 ounces
- Barbecue sauce - .75 cup
- Liquid smoke - .5 teaspoon
- Red cabbage, shredded – 1.5 cups
- Carrots, shredded - .5 cup
- Red onion, diced - .5 cup
- Date sugar - .5 teaspoon
- Sea salt – 1.5 teaspoons
- Apple cider vinegar – 1 tablespoon
- Garlic powder - .5 teaspoon
- Mayonnaise 2 tablespoons
- Black pepper, ground - .25 teaspoon
- Whole wheat buns - 4

**Directions:**

1. Place the sliced tempeh in a glass baking dish and coat it in the barbecue sauce and the liquid smoke. While you don't have to add the liquid smoke, it is a great

addition that makes it taste as if it has come freshly off the grill. Allow the dish to marinate for at least forty-five minutes.

2. When the tempeh is nearly done marinating begin to preheat your oven to Fahrenheit four-hundred and fifty degrees.

3. Cover the tempeh in a sheet of aluminum and allow it to bake for first thirty minutes, and then remove the aluminum and bake it for an additional five minutes.

4. Meanwhile, prepare the slaw by combining the remaining ingredients (except for the buns) in a bowl. Once combined, cover the bowl and allow it to meld in the fridge until the tempeh is done cooking. It is best to make the slaw when you first put the tempeh in the oven, rather than near the end, as it gives the flavors longer to meld.

5. To serve divide the tempeh strips between the buns and then top them off with the slaw.

**Nutrition:** Calories: 382

# Tofu Tikka Masala

**Preparation Time: 10 minutes**

**Cooking Time: 25 minutes**

**Servings: 4**

**Ingredients:**

- Tofu, extra-firm, sliced into bite-sized cubes – 14 ounces
- Cumin – 1 teaspoon
- Ginger, peeled and grated – 2 teaspoons
- Sweet paprika - .5 teaspoon
- Turmeric - .5 teaspoon
- Garlic, minced – 2 cloves
- Garam masala – 1.5 teaspoons
- Coriander powder - .5 teaspoon
- Cayenne - .25 teaspoon
- Tomato passata (if not available use puree) – 1 cup
- Coconut milk, full-fat – 14 ounces
- Olive oil – 2 tablespoons
- Red onion, diced – 1
- Sea salt – 1 teaspoon

**Directions:**

1. Add the olive oil, red onion, and salt to a skillet and allow it to cook over medium until the onions have become soft, about five minutes. Add in the grated ginger and minced garlic, cooking for a minute before adding in all the spices. Cook for an additional two minutes, until the spices are fragrant. Keep a close eye on the spices, stirring constantly to avoid burning.

2. Stir the tomato passata or puree into the skillet and allow it to continue cooking until thickened and reduced, about ten to fifteen minutes.

3. Add the tofu and canned coconut milk to the skillet and bring the pan to a boil. Reduce the stove to low and allow the tikka masala to simmer for ten minutes. Serve warm over brown rice or buckwheat.

**Nutrition:** Calories: 344

# Tempeh Vegan Chili

**Preparation Time: 10 minutes**

**Cooking Time: 20 minutes**

**Servings: 4**

**Ingredients:**

- Tempeh, roughly grated – 8 ounces
- Extra virgin olive oil – 2 tablespoons
- Red onion, diced – 1
- Celery, diced – 1 rib
- Bell pepper, diced – 1
- Garlic, minced – 4 cloves
- Black beans, drained and rinsed – 15 ounces
- Kidney beans, drained and rinsed – 15 ounces
- Tomato sauce - .75 cup
- Water – 1.25 cups
- Chili powder - 1 tablespoon
- Crushed red pepper flakes - .25 teaspoon
- Cumin, ground – 2 teaspoons
- Sea salt – 1 teaspoon
- Cocoa powder – 1 tablespoon

**Directions:**

1. Add the extra virgin olive oil and grated tempeh to a large pot and allow it to brown over medium heat for five minutes.

2. Add the celery, garlic, bell pepper, and onions to the pot, cooking until slightly tender, about five more minutes.

3. Stir in the remaining ingredient and allow the chili to simmer and the flavors to meld for approximately fifteen more minutes. Serve warm with your favorite chili toppings.

**Nutrition:** Calories: 455

# Eggroll in a Bowl

**Preparation Time: 10 minutes**

**Cooking Time: 15 minutes**

**Servings: 6**

**Ingredients:**

- Chicken broth - .25 cup

- Extra virgin olive oil – 2 tablespoon, divided

- Ground turkey – 1 pound

- Garlic, minced – 3 cloves

- Red cabbage, shredded – 5 cups

- Ginger, minced - .5 teaspoon

- Carrots, shredded – 1 cup

- Onion, finely diced – 1.5 cups

- Sea salt - .5 teaspoon

- Sesame seed oil – 1 teaspoon

- Apple cider vinegar – 2 teaspoons

- Tamari sauce – 2 tablespoons

- Black pepper, ground - .25 teaspoon

**Directions:**

1. Add one tablespoon of the extra virgin olive oil to a large pot and brown the ground turkey over medium

---

heat until cooked nearly all the way cooked through, about five minutes.

2. Push the turkey to the side of the pan and then add the remaining olive oil and the diced onion to the center. Sauté the onion until translucent, about five minutes. Stir in the ginger, garlic, and carrots, cooking for two minutes until fragrant. Stir the vegetables and turkey all together.

3. Pour the chicken broth into the large pot and scrape the bottom of the pot with a wooden spoon to deglaze it.

4. Stir in the sea salt, tamari sauce, red cabbage, and ground pepper until well combined. Cover the pot with a lid and reduce the heat to medium-low. Continue cooking the ingredients until the red cabbage is tender, about twelve to fifteen minutes.

5. Remove the large pot from the heat of the stove and stir in the sesame seed oil. Serve alone, or with the Egg Fried Buckwheat from the side dish chapter.

**Nutrition:** Calories: 208

# Beef and Red Cabbage Soup

**Preparation Time:** 10 minutes

**Cooking Time:** 35 minutes

**Servings:** 6

**Ingredients:**

- Beef broth – 4 cups
- Fire roasted crushed tomatoes – 28 ounces
- Ground beef – 1 pound
- Celery, chopped – 2 stalks
- Onion, diced – 1
- Carrot, chopped – 1
- Bell pepper, diced – 1
- Garlic, minced – 3 cloves
- Red cabbage, chopped – 1 head
- Sea salt – 1.5 teaspoons
- Italian herb seasoning – 1 tablespoon
- Fresh thyme – 2 sprigs
- Spicy brown mustard – 1 tablespoon
- Black pepper, ground - .25 teaspoon

**Directions:**

1. Add the ground beef to a large steel soup pot and brown it over medium-high heat until fully cooked. Once done cooking, drain off most of the excess fat, leaving only about two tablespoons in the pot. Set the ground beef aside.

2. Into the now empty soup pot add the reserved beef fat along with the carrot, celery, onion, and bell pepper. Cook until the vegetables are tender, about six minutes. Add in the garlic and cook until fragrant, about one more minute.

3. Return the cooked ground beef to the soup pot along with the beef broth, crushed tomatoes, seasonings, and spicy brown mustard, stirring it all together to combine. Bring the pot of beef and tomatoes to a boil and then reduce to a simmer, cooking for fifteen to twenty minutes.

4. Stir the cabbage into the soup, allowing it to cook until tender, about ten to fifteen minutes. Serve alone or over either cooked rice or buckwheat.

**Nutrition:** Calories: 362

# Parmesan Chicken and Kale Sauté

**Preparation Time:** 10 minutes

**Cooking Time:** 15 minutes

**Servings:** 6

**Ingredients:**

- Chicken breasts, boneless and skinless – 1.5 pounds

- Extra virgin olive oil – 2 tablespoon

- Sea salt – 1 teaspoon

- Onion, diced – 1

- Red pepper flakes - .25 teaspoon

- Lemon juice – 1 tablespoon

- Black pepper, ground - .25 teaspoon

- Garlic, minced – 3 cloves

- Chicken broth – .5 cup

- Parmesan cheese, grated - .5 cup

- Kale, chopped – 12 ounces

**Directions:**

1. Slice the chicken breasts into long strips, each half an inch thick.

2. Add the extra virgin olive oil to a large skillet and set the stove to medium heat. Allow the olive oil to heat until it shimmers, but don't let it smoke. Add the

chicken, sea salt, and black pepper, sautéing it until the chicken is fully cooked through, about five to seven minutes. The chicken breasts are ready when they reaches an internal temperature of Fahrenheit one-hundred and sixty-five degrees.

3. Transfer the cooked chicken breast to a plate and cover it with aluminum or a lid to keep it warm.

4. Add the minced garlic, diced onion, and red pepper flakes to the now empty skillet, sautéing for about two minutes until the onions soften.

5. Add the kale and broth to the skillet and then cover with a lid. Stir occasionally, allowing the kale to cook until tender, about five minutes.

6. Add the cooked chicken breast back into the skillet along with the lemon juice and Parmesan cheese. Stir everything to combine and then remove the skillet from the heat before serving.

**Nutrition:** Calories: 361

# Parsley Pesto Pasta

**Preparation Time:** 10 minutes

**Cooking Time:** 15 minutes

**Servings:** 5

**Ingredients:**

- Parsley, fresh, packed – 2 cups
- Garlic – 3 cloves
- Pine nuts - .25 cup
- Sea salt – 1 teaspoon
- Lemon juice – 2 tablespoons
- Coconut cream – 5 tablespoons
- Nutritional yeast – 3 tablespoons
- Black pepper, ground - .25 teaspoon
- Almonds - .5 cup
- Nutritional yeast – 1 tablespoon
- Sea salt - .25 teaspoon
- Pasta of choice – 200 grams

**Directions:**

1. In a food processor mix together the parsley, garlic, pine nuts, teaspoon of sea salt, lemon juice, coconut cream, three tablespoons of nutritional yeast, and the

black pepper to create the parsley pesto. Scrape down the sides of the food processor as needed.

2. In a blender combine the almonds and one tablespoon of nutritional yeast until it forms a fine meal. This will be your vegan Parmesan cheese.

3. Meanwhile, cook the pasta according to the instructions on the packaging until it is al dente. Drain the water off of the cooked pasta and return it back to the pot.

4. Pour the pesto over the pasta and allow it to cook together over medium heat while constantly stirring for one to two minutes. Remove the pot from the heat.

5. Serve the pasta, topping it off with the vegan Parmesan cheese you previously prepared.

**Nutrition:** Calories: 348 Carbohydrates: 7.4 g Cholesterol: 44 mg Fat: 3.2 g

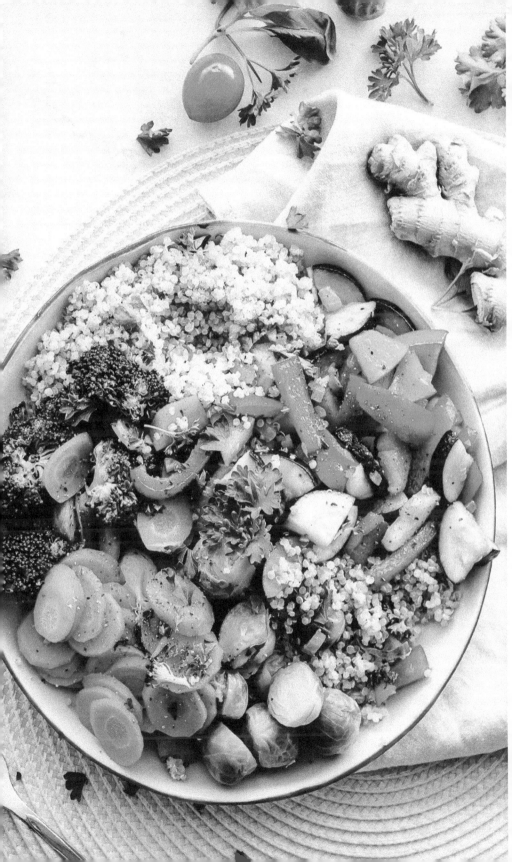

# SIRTFOOD VEGETABLES

# Parsley Butter Asparagus

**Preparation Time:** 10 minutes

**Cooking time:** 15 minutes

**Servings:** 4

**Ingredients:**

- 9 oz asparagus
- ¼ cup fresh parsley, chopped
- 2 tablespoons butter
- 1 teaspoon ground paprika
- ½ teaspoon salt
- 1 cup water, for cooking

**Directions:**

1. Pour water in the pan and bring it to boil.
2. Meanwhile, trim the asparagus and cut into the halves.
3. Put the prepared asparagus in the boiling water and boil for 5 minutes.
4. Then drain water and chill asparagus in the ice water.
5. Toss butter in the saucepan. Melt it.
6. Add chilled asparagus and stir gently. When the asparagus is coated in the butter, sprinkle it with ground paprika and salt.

7. Close the lid and cook the side dish for 10 minutes over the medium-low heat.

**Nutrition:** calories 67, fat 5.9, fiber 1.7, carbs 3, protein 1.7

# Baked Bell Peppers with Oil Dressing

**Preparation Time: 10 minutes**

**Cooking time: 10 minutes**

**Servings:2**

**Ingredients:**

- 8 oz green bell peppers (appx.4 bell peppers)
- 4 tablespoons olive oil
- ½ teaspoon minced garlic
- ¼ teaspoon chili flakes
- ½ teaspoon dried cilantro
- ½ teaspoon paprika
- ½ teaspoon salt

**Directions:**

1. Pierce the bell peppers with the help of knife and place in the tray.
2. Bake the peppers for 10 minutes at 385F. Flip the peppers onto another side after 5 minutes of cooking.
3. Meanwhile, make oil dressing: whisk together olive oil, minced garlic, chili flakes, dried cilantro, paprika, and salt.
4. When the bell peppers are baked, remove them from the oven and chill little.

5. Then peel the peppers and clean from the seeds.

6. Sprinkle the bell peppers with the oil dressing and mix up gently.

**Nutrition:** calories 267, fat 28.3, fiber 2.2, carbs 6.1 protein 1.2

# Cauliflower Cakes

**Preparation Time:** 15 minutes

**Cooking time:** 7 minutes

**Servings:** 5

**Ingredients:**

- 1 cup cauliflower, shredded
- 1 egg, beaten
- 5 oz Swiss cheese, shredded
- 2 tablespoons almond flour
- ½ teaspoon ground black pepper
- ¼ teaspoon salt
- 1 tablespoon avocado oil

**Directions:**

1. Place the shredded cauliflower and beaten egg in the big bowl.
2. Sprinkle the ingredients with shredded cheese.
3. Then add almond flour, ground black pepper, and salt.
4. With the help of the spoon mix up the mass well.
5. When it is homogenous and smooth – the cauliflower mixture is ready.
6. Pour avocado oil in the skillet and preheat it until it starts to boil.

7. Make the small cauliflower cakes with the help of the big spoon and place them in the hot skillet.

8. Press the cakes little and roast them for 3 minutes from each side.

9. When the cauliflower cakes get light brown color, transfer them in the plate. Dry them with the paper towel if needed.

**Nutrition:** calories 194, fat 14.7, fiber 1.9, carbs 5.4, protein 11.6

# Vegetable Plate

**Preparation Time: 10 minutes**

**Cooking time: 40 minutes**

**Servings:9**

**Ingredients:**

- 1/3 cup cherry tomatoes
- 2 bell peppers
- 1 eggplant, trimmed
- 1 zucchini, trimmed
- 1/3 cup okra, trimmed
- 1 tablespoon butter
- 1 tablespoon sesame oil
- 1 tablespoon fresh rosemary
- 1 teaspoon salt
- 1 teaspoon chili flakes
- ½ teaspoon ground nutmeg

**Directions:**

1. Slice the eggplant and zucchini roughly and transfer them in the tray.
2. Chop the okra roughly and add in the tray too.
3. Then add cherry tomatoes, bell peppers, and mix up the vegetables with the help of the hand palms gently.

4. Sprinkle the vegetables with the sesame oil, fresh rosemary, salt, chili flakes, ground nutmeg, and add butter.

5. Mix up the vegetables one more time.

6. Preheat the oven to 365F.

7. Place the tray with the vegetables in the oven and cook for 40 minutes.

8. Mix up the vegetables with the help of the spatula from time to time.

9. Nutrition: calories 54, fat 3.1, fiber 2.8, carbs 6.6, protein 1.2

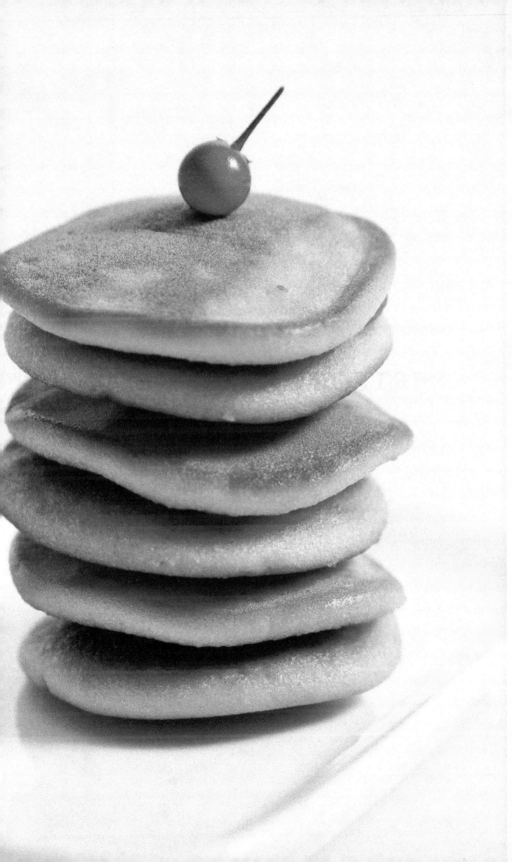

# SIRTFOOD SNACK RECIPES

# Potato Bites

**Preparation Time: 10 minutes**

**Cooking Time: 20 minutes**

**Servings: 3**

**Ingredients:**

- 1 potato, sliced
- 2 bacon slices, already cooked and crumbled
- 1 small avocado, pitted and cubed
- Cooking spray

**Directions:**

1. Spread potato slices on a lined baking sheet, spray with cooking oil, introduce in the oven at 350 degrees F, bake for 20 minutes, arrange on a platter, top each slice with avocado and crumbled bacon and serve as a snack.
2. Enjoy!

**Nutrition:** Calories: 180 Fat: 4g Fiber: 1g Carbohydrates: 8g Protein: 6g

# Sesame Dip

**Preparation Time:** 10 minutes

**Cooking Time:** 0 minutes

**Servings:** 6

**Ingredients:**

- 1 cup sesame seed paste, pure
- Black pepper to the taste
- 1 cup veggie stock
- ½ cup lemon juice
- ½ teaspoon cumin, ground
- 3 garlic cloves, chopped

**Directions:**

1. In your food processor, mix the sesame paste with black pepper, stock, lemon juice, cumin and garlic, pulse very well, divide into bowls and serve as a party dip.
2. Enjoy!
3. Nutrition: calories 120, fat 12, fiber 2, carbs 7, protein 4
4. Rosemary Squash Dip
5. Preparation time: 10 minutes
6. Cooking time: 40 minutes
7. Servings: 4

**Nutrition:** Calories: 182 Fat: 5g Fiber: 7g Carbohydrates: 12g Protein: 5g

# Bean Spread

**Preparation Time:** 10 minutes

**Cooking Time:** 6 hours

**Servings:** 4

**Ingredients:**

- 1 cup white beans, dried
- 1 teaspoon apple cider vinegar
- 1 cup veggie stock
- 1 tablespoon water

**Directions:**

1. In your slow cooker, mix beans with stock, stir, cover, cook on Low for 6 hours, drain, transfer to your food processor, add vinegar and water, pulse well, divide into bowls and serve.

2. Enjoy!

**Nutrition:** Calories: 181 Fat: 6 Fiber: 5 Carbohydrates: 9 Protein: 7

# Eggplant Salsa

**Preparation Time:** 10 minutes

**Cooking Time:** 10 minutes

**Servings:** 4

**Ingredients:**

- 1 and ½ cups tomatoes, chopped
- 3 cups eggplant, cubed
- A drizzle of olive oil
- 2 teaspoons capers
- 6 ounces green olives, pitted and sliced
- 4 garlic cloves, minced
- 2 teaspoons balsamic vinegar
- 1 tablespoon basil, chopped
- Black pepper to the taste

**Directions:**

1. Heat up a pan with the oil over medium-high heat, add eggplant, stir and cook for 5 minutes.
2. Add tomatoes, capers, olives, garlic, vinegar, basil and black pepper, toss, cook for 5 minutes more, divide into small cups and serve cold.
3. Enjoy!

**Nutrition:** Calories: 120 Fat: 6g Fiber: 5g Carbohydrates: 9g Protein: 7g

# Carrots and Cauliflower Spread

**Preparation Time:** 10 minutes

**Cooking Time:** 40 minutes

**Servings:** 4

**Ingredients:**

- 1 cup carrots, sliced
- 2 cups cauliflower florets
- ½ cup cashews
- 2 and ½ cups water
- 1 cup almond milk
- 1 teaspoon garlic powder
- ¼ teaspoon smoked paprika

**Directions:**

1. In a small pot, mix the carrots with cauliflower, cashews and water, stir, cover, bring to a boil over medium heat, cook for 40 minutes, drain and transfer to a blender.
2. Add almond milk, garlic powder and paprika, pulse well, divide into small bowls and serve
3. Enjoy!

**Nutrition:** Calories: 201 Fat: 7g Fiber: 4g Carbohydrates: 7gProtein: 7g

# Italian Veggie Salsa

**Preparation Time:** 10 minutes

**Cooking Time:** 10 minutes

**Servings:** 4

**Ingredients:**

- 2 red bell peppers, cut into medium wedges
- 3 zucchinis, sliced
- ½ cup garlic, minced
- 2 tablespoons olive oil
- A pinch of black pepper
- 1 teaspoon Italian seasoning

**Directions:**

1. Heat up a pan with the oil over medium-high heat, add bell peppers and zucchini, toss and cook for 5 minutes.
2. Add garlic, black pepper and Italian seasoning, toss, cook for 5 minutes more, divide into small cups and serve as a snack.
3. Enjoy!

**Nutrition:** Calories: 132 Fat: 3g Fiber: 3g Carbohydrates: 7g Protein: 4g

# Black Bean Salsa

**Preparation Time:** 10 minutes

**Cooking Time:** 0 minutes

**Servings:** 6

**Ingredients:**

- 1 tablespoon coconut aminos
- ½ teaspoon cumin, ground
- 1 cup canned black beans, no-salt-added, drained and rinsed
- 1 cup salsa
- 6 cups romaine lettuce leaves, torn
- ½ cup avocado, peeled, pitted and cubed

**Directions:**

1. In a bowl, combine the beans with the aminos, cumin, salsa, lettuce and avocado, toss, divide into small bowls and serve as a snack.
2. Enjoy!

**Nutrition:** Calories: 181 Fat: 4g Fiber: 7g Carbohydrates: 14g Protein: 7g

# Corn Spread

**Preparation Time: 10 minutes**

**Cooking Time: 10 minutes**

**Servings: 6**

**Ingredients:**

- 30 ounces canned corn, drained
- 2 green onions, chopped
- ½ cup coconut cream
- 1 jalapeno, chopped
- ½ teaspoon chili powder

**Directions:**

1. In a small pan, combine the corn with green onions, jalapeno and chili powder, stir, bring to a simmer, cook over medium heat for 10 minutes, leave aside to cool down, add coconut cream, stir well, divide into small bowls and serve as a spread.

2. Enjoy!

**Nutrition:** Calories: 192 Fat: 5g Fiber: 10g Carbs: 11g Protein: 8g

# Mushroom Dip

**Preparation Time: 10 minutes**

**Cooking Time: 20 minutes**

**Servings: 6**

**Ingredients:**

- 1 cup yellow onion, chopped
- 3 garlic cloves, minced
- 1 pound mushrooms, chopped
- 28 ounces tomato sauce, no-salt-added
- Black pepper to the taste

**Directions:**

1. Put the onion in a pot, add garlic, mushrooms, black pepper and tomato sauce, stir, cook over medium heat for 20 minutes, leave aside to cool down, divide into small bowls and serve.
2. Enjoy!

**Nutrition:** Calories 215 Fat: 4g Fiber: 7g Carbs: 3g Protein: 7g

# Salsa Bean Dip

**Preparation Time:** 10 minutes

**Cooking Time:** 20 minutes

**Servings:** 6

**Ingredients:**

- ½ cup salsa
- 2 cups canned white beans, no-salt-added, drained and rinsed
- 1 cup low-fat cheddar, shredded
- 2 tablespoons green onions, chopped

**Directions:**

1. In a small pot, combine the beans with the green onions and salsa, stir, bring to a simmer over medium heat, cook for 20 minutes, add cheese, stir until it melts, take off heat, leave aside to cool down, divide into bowls and serve.
2. Enjoy!

**Nutrition:** Calories: 212g Fat: 5g Fiber: 6g Carbs: 10g Protein: 8g Mung Sprouts Salsa Preparation time: 10 minutes Cooking time: 0 minutes Servings: 2

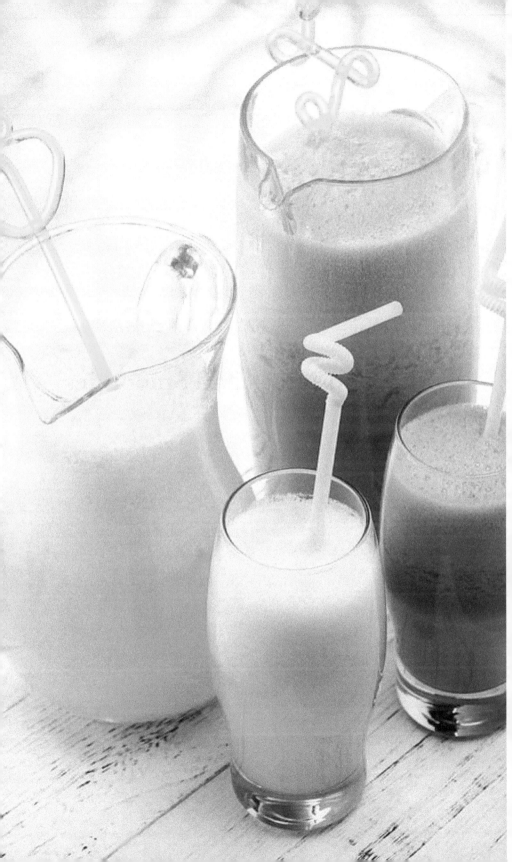

# Sirtfood Juices and Smoothies

# Sirt Food Cocktail

**Preparation Time:** 5 minutes

**Cooking Time:** 0 minute

**Servings:** 1

**Ingredients:**

- 75g (3oz) kale

- 50g (2oz) strawberries

- 1 apple, cored

- 2 sticks of celery

- 1 tablespoon parsley

- 1 teaspoon of matcha powder

**Directions:**

1. Place the ingredients into a blender and add enough water to cover the ingredients and blitz to a smooth consistency.

2. Squeeze lemon juice (optional) to taste

**Nutrition:** Calories: 101

# Summer Berry Smoothie

**Preparation Time:** 7 minutes

**Cooking Time:** 0 minute

**Servings:** 1

**Ingredients:**

- 50g (2oz) blueberries
- 50g (2oz) strawberries
- 25g (1oz) blackcurrants
- 25g (1oz) red grapes
- 1 carrot, peeled
- 1 orange, peeled
- Juice of 1 lime

**Directions:**

1. Place all of the ingredients into a blender and cover them with water. Blitz until smooth. You can also add some crushed ice and a mint leaf to garnish.

**Nutrition:** Calories: 146

# Mango, Celery & Ginger Smoothie

**Preparation Time: 5 minutes**

**Cooking Time: 0 minute**

**Servings: 1**

**Ingredients:**

- 1 stalk of celery
- 50g (2oz) kale
- 1 apple, cored
- 50g (2oz) mango, peeled, de-stoned and chopped
- 2.5cm (1 inch) chunk of fresh ginger root, peeled and chopped

**Directions:**

1. Put all the ingredients into a blender with some water and blitz until smooth. Add ice to make your smoothie really refreshing.

**Nutrition:** Calories: 105

# Orange, Carrot & Kale Smoothie

**Preparation Time:** 7 minutes

**Cooking Time:** 0 minute

**Servings:** 1

**Ingredients:**

- 1 carrot, peeled

- 1 orange, peeled

- 1 stick of celery

- 1 apple, cored

- 50g (2oz) kale

- ½ teaspoon matcha powder

**Directions:**

1. Place all of the ingredients into a blender and add in enough water to cover them. Process until smooth, serve and enjoy.

**Nutrition:** Calories: 156

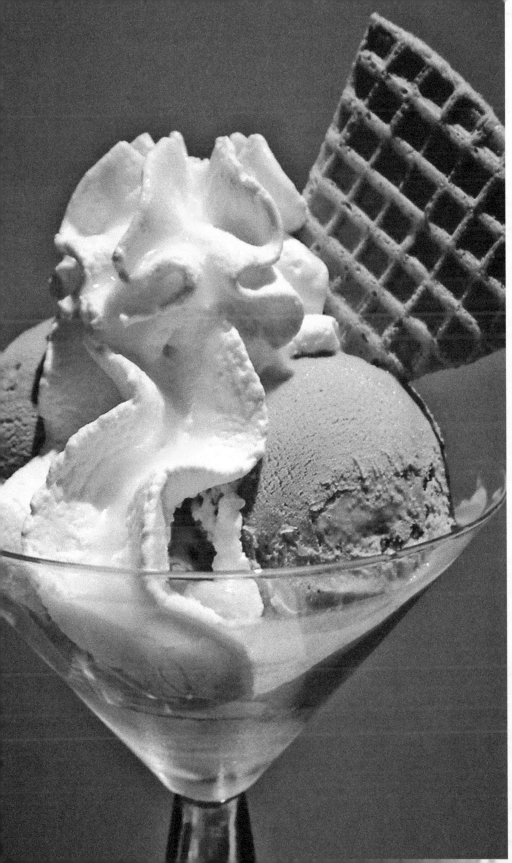

# Sirt Desserts

# Choc Nut Truffles

**Preparation Time:** 10 minutes

**Cooking Time:** 15 minutes

**Servings:** 1

**Ingredients:**

- 150g 5oz desiccated shredded coconut
- 50g 2oz walnuts, chopped
- 25g 1oz hazelnuts, chopped
- 4 Medrol dates
- 2 tablespoons 100% cocoa powder or cacao nibs
- 1 tablespoon coconut oil

**Directions:**

1. Place ingredients into a blender and process until smooth and creamy. Using a teaspoon, scoop the mixture into bite-size pieces then roll it into balls. Place them into small paper cases, cover them and chill for 1 hour before serving.

**Nutrition:** Calories: 236

# No-Bake Strawberry Flapjacks

**Preparation Time:** 10 minutes

**Cooking Time:** 15 minutes

**Servings:** 1

**Ingredients:**

- 75g 3oz porridge oats
- 125g 4oz dates
- 50g 2oz strawberries
- 50g 2oz peanuts unsalted
- 50g 2oz walnuts
- 1 tablespoon coconut oil
- 2 tablespoons 100% cocoa powder or cacao nibs

**Directions:**

1. Place ingredients into a blender and process until they become a soft consistency. Spread the mixture onto a baking sheet or small flat tin. Press the mixture down and smooth it out. Cut it into 8 pieces, ready to serve. You can add an extra sprinkling of cocoa powder to garnish if you wish.

**Nutrition:** 182 calories each

# Chocolate Balls

**Preparation Time:** 10 minutes

**Cooking Time:** 15 minutes

**Servings:** 1

**Ingredients:**

- 50g 2oz peanut butter or almond butter
- 25g 1oz cocoa powder
- 25g 1oz desiccated shredded coconut
- 1 tablespoon honey
- 1 tablespoon cocoa powder for coating

**Directions:**

1. Mix all ingredients into a bowl. Scoop out a little of the mixture and shape it into a ball. Roll the ball in a little cocoa powder and set aside. Repeat for the remaining mixture. Can be eaten straight away or stored in the fridge.

**Nutrition:** 115 calories per serving

# Warm Berries & Cream

**Preparation Time:** 10 minutes

**Cooking Time:** 15 minutes

**Servings:** 1

**Ingredients:**

- 250g 9oz blueberries
- 250g 9oz strawberries
- 100g 3½ oz. redcurrants
- 100g 3½ oz. blackberries
- 4 tablespoons fresh whipped cream
- 1 tablespoon honey

**Directions:**

1. Mix all ingredients into a bowl. Scoop out a little of the mixture and shape it into a ball. Roll the ball in a little cocoa powder and set aside. Repeat for the remaining mixture. Can be eaten straight away or stored in the fridge.

**Nutrition:** 115 calories per serving

# CONCLUSION

Time and time once again, I've explained to you guys the problem with the majority of diets: restrictive consuming. When it pertains to constraint, our rebel impulses desire to stick it to the guy and binge like crazy. I'm quite sure you'll also become that good friend that nobody desires to go out with because of your brand-new hangry character. For realists, there have not been sufficient constant research studies that say calorie limitation is the way to go. You'll lose some sweet however you'll also fulfill some undesirable outcomes and ultimately restore the weight. Research studies looking at caloric constraint discovered that in time limitation results in loss of muscle mass (which completely counters what the sirtfood diet plan claims it can do), muscle strength and loss of bone, anemia, depression, and irritation.

The most significant claim this diet boasts about is these sirtuin proteins increase our body's ability to burn fat, promote muscle repair work, growth and upkeep and as pointed out earlier- quick weight-loss. Right?! Because rapid weight loss is always safe. Other non-weight associated advantages consist of: improving memory, managing blood sugar level levels, and protecting you from cancers and persistent illness.

The Sirtfood diet stresses consuming foods that might engage with a household of proteins known to be as sirtuin proteins (now the name of the diet plan is starting to make sense). Since of the role they play in the metabolic process, some professionals are calling sirtuins "slim genes" for their prospective function in weight loss.

Sirtfoods promote sirtuin genes, which are stated to influence the body's capability to burn fat and boost the metabolic system.

The Sirtfood diet plan is based upon 2 stages:

Phase one is an intensive seven-day program developed to kick-start your intense weight reduction.

Then stage 2 has to do with upping the amount of Sirtfood-rich fruit and vegetables in your everyday meals to preserve weight-loss.

Unlike numerous short-term diets, the Sirtfood plan includes meals and guidance on how to keep off the weight you lose in the very first week by continuing to incorporate Sirtfoods as part of a well-balanced and healthy diet plan

CPSIA information can be obtained
at www.ICGtesting.com
Printed in the USA
BVHW012049300721
613019BV00040B/578